# Table of Contents

Diabetes is a chronic condition that affects millions of people worldwide. It is a disease that occurs when the body is unable to regulate blood sugar levels properly. High blood sugar levels can lead to a range of health problems, including heart disease, kidney disease, nerve damage, and blindness.

Type 1 diabetes is an autoimmune disease that occurs when the body attacks and destroys the insulin-producing cells in the pancreas. This results in the body not being able to produce enough insulin to regulate blood sugar levels. Type 1 diabetes is usually diagnosed in children and young adults.

Type 2 diabetes, on the other hand, is a condition in which the body becomes resistant to insulin or does not produce enough insulin to regulate blood sugar levels. Type 2 diabetes is more common than type 1 diabetes, and it is usually diagnosed in adults.

Gestational diabetes is a type of diabetes that occurs during pregnancy. This type of diabetes usually goes away after the baby is born, but it can increase the risk of developing type 2 diabetes later in life.

## The Importance of a Healthy Diet for Diabetics

Diabetes is a condition that affects the way the body processes glucose, which is the primary source of energy for the body's cells. In a healthy individual, glucose is regulated by the hormone insulin, which is produced by the pancreas. In a person with diabetes, however, the body is either unable to produce insulin (Type 1 diabetes) or cannot use it properly (Type 2 diabetes). As a result, glucose builds up in the bloodstream, leading to a range of health complications.

One of the key ways to manage diabetes is through diet. A healthy diet can help regulate blood sugar levels, reduce the risk of complications, and improve overall health. For diabetics, it's important to choose foods that are low in sugar, low in fat, and high in fiber. This can help keep blood sugar levels stable, reduce the risk of heart disease, and help manage weight.

Foods that are high in sugar should be avoided, as they can cause blood sugar levels to spike. This includes sweets, desserts, and sugary drinks. Instead, diabetics should focus on eating fruits and vegetables, whole grains, lean proteins, and low-fat dairy products. These foods are high in fiber, which can help regulate blood sugar levels and keep diabetics feeling full and satisfied.

In addition to making healthy food choices, diabetics should also pay attention to portion sizes. Eating too much of any type of food can cause blood sugar levels to rise. By keeping portion sizes moderate, diabetics can help manage their blood sugar levels and maintain a healthy weight.

Grilled goat's cheese with cranberry dressing

Ingredients

2 red-skinned apples

3 tbsp lemon juice

3 x Capricorn goat's cheese, halved horizontally

2 tbsp cranberry jelly

2 tbsp olive oil

1 tsp clear honey

25g pecan

2 chicory heads, separated into leaves

handful radish  sprouts (available  from  larger  supermarkets)  or watercress

Method

STEP 1

Quarter, core, then thinly slice the apple into a bowl with the lemon juice and 1 tbsp water. Toss well, as this stops the apples going brown.

STEP 2

Heat grill to high, then line your grill rack with foil. Put the cheeses rind-side down on the foil, then set aside for a moment.

STEP 3

Drain 2 tbsp of the juice from the apple bowl into another small bowl and discard the rest. Add the cranberry sauce, oil and honey with some seasoning, and whisk to form a dressing. Grill the cheeses for 4 mins, then scatter the nuts on and around the cheeses and return to the grill to cook for a few mins more – but take care that the nuts don't burn.

STEP 4

Arrange the apple, chicory and radish sprouts or watercress on 6 plates, then carefully top with the hot melted cheese. Scatter over the nuts, spoon over the dressing and serve straight away.

Low-fat roasties

Ingredients

800g roasting potatoes, quartered

1 garlic clove, sliced

200ml vegetable stock (from a cube is fine)

2 tbsp olive oil

Method

STEP 1

Heat oven to 200C/fan 180C/gas 6. Put the potatoes and garlic in a roasting tin. Pour over the stock, then brush the tops of the potatoes with half the olive oil. Season, then cook for 50 mins. Brush with the remaining oil and cook 10-15 mins more until the stock is absorbed and the potatoes have browned and cooked through.

Juicy Lucy pudding

Ingredients

350g packet frozen fruits of the forest, defrosted

3 tbsp light muscovado sugar

4 tbsp no-added-sugar wild blueberry jam (we used St Dalfour, from larger supermarket branches)

6 medium-sized ripe pears, peeled, quartered and cored

50g fresh white breadcrumb

25g butter, melted

Method

STEP 1

Preheat the oven to 190C/gas 5/ fan 170C. Mix the fruits of the forest in a large bowl with the sugar and jam, then add the pears and toss to mix. Tip into a deep baking dish measuring about 18x28cm, cover with foil and roast in the oven for 20 minutes. Pierce a pear or two to see if they are really tender; if not, return dish to the oven for another 5 minutes or until they feel soft.

STEP 2

Mix breadcrumbs with the butter and scatter over the fruit. Bake uncovered in the oven for 10-15 minutes or until golden and crispy. Serve hot.

Chargrilled vegetable salad

Ingredients

2 red peppers

3 tbsp olive oil

1 tbsp red wine vinegar

1 small garlic clove, crushed

1 red chilli, deseeded, finely chopped

1 aubergine, cut into 1cm rounds

2 red onions, sliced about 1.5cm thick but kept as whole slices

6 plump sundried tomatoes in oil, drained and torn into strips

handful black olives

large handful basil, roughly torn

Method

STEP 1

First, blacken the peppers all over – do this directly over a flame, over hot coals or under a hot grill. When completely blackened, put them in a bowl, cover with a plate and leave to cool.

STEP 2

While the peppers are cooling, mix the oil, vinegar, garlic and chilli in a large bowl. On a hot barbecue or griddle pan, chargrill the aubergine, courgette and onions in batches until they have defined grill marks on both sides and are starting to soften. The time will depend on the intensity of your grill, so use your judgement – courgettes and red onions are fine still slightly crunchy but you want the aubergine cooked all the way through. As the vegetables are ready, put them straight into the dressing to marinate, breaking the onions up into rings.

STEP 3

When the peppers are cool enough to handle, peel, remove the stalk and scrape out the seeds. Cut into strips and toss through the veg with any juice from the bowl. Mix in the tomatoes, olives, basil and seasoning. Drizzle with more oil, if you like, and serve either on its own or with mozzarella or crumbled feta.

Turkey & parsnip curry

Ingredients

2 tbsp vegetable oil

2 onions, halved through the root and thinly sliced

500g parsnip, peeled and cut into chunks

5 tbsp Madras curry paste

400g can chopped tomatoes

500g/1lb 2oz boneless cooked turkey, cut into chunks

150g pot low-fat natural yogurt

cooked basmati rice, to serve

Method

STEP 1

Heat the oil in a saucepan, add the onions and fry gently for 10 minutes until they are softened and lightly coloured. Add the parsnips and stir well.

STEP 2

To make the curry, stir in the curry paste, then add the tomatoes with a little salt, and stir well. Add 1½ canfuls of water and bring to the boil. Reduce the heat, cover and simmer for 15-20 minutes, until the parsnips are just tender.

STEP 3

To finish, stir in the turkey chunks, cover the pan again and simmer for a further 5 minutes until the turkey is heated through. Remove from the heat. (The curry can now be cooled and frozen for up to 2 months.) Lightly swirl in the yogurt and serve with basmati rice.

Chargrilled fish with green chilli, coriander and coconut relish

Ingredients

1 small red onion, finely chopped

1 tsp finely grated fresh ginger

1 tsp mustard seeds

20g (1/4 cup) shredded coconut

1 truss tomato, seeded, finely chopped

1 long fresh green chilli, seeded, thinly sliced

1/4 cup chopped fresh coriander

1 tbsp lime juice

Pinch of caster sugar

4 (about 150g each) firm white fish fillets

Steamed green beans, to serve

Steamed asparagus, to serve

Methods

Step 1

Heat a frying pan over medium heat. Spray with oil. Stir in the onion for 5 minutes or until soft. Stir in the ginger and mustard seeds for 30 seconds or until aromatic. Stir in the coconut for 1-2 minutes or until light golden. Transfer to a bowl. Set aside to cool slightly. Stir in the tomato, chilli, coriander, lime juice and sugar.

Step 2

Preheat a barbecue grill or chargrill on high. Spray the fish with oil. Cook on grill for 2-3 minutes each side or until golden and fish flakes easily when tested with a fork.

Step 3

Divide the steamed vegetables among plates. Top with the fish and a spoonful of the coconut mixture.

Roast pork with couscous & ginger yogurt

Ingredients

2 pork fillets, each about 500g/1lb 2oz, trimmed of any fat

2 tsp olive oil

3 tsp ground cumin

1 tsp ground cinnamon

4 tsp grated ginger

250g couscous

100g sultanas

zest and juice 1 lemon

small bunch mint, chopped

200g fat-free natural yogurt


Method

STEP 1

Heat oven to 190C/170C fan/gas 5. Brown the pork in a non-stick frying pan over a high heat for 4-5 mins, turning twice. Mix the oil, 2 tsp cumin, cinnamon, 2 tsp ginger and some seasoning, then rub all over the pork. Transfer to a roasting tin and roast for 30-35 mins or until the juices run clear when the thickest part is pierced with a skewer.

STEP 2

Mix the couscous with the remaining cumin, the sultanas, lemon zest and juice, then season and pour over 400ml boiling water. Stir well and cover for 5 mins, then stir in the mint.

STEP 3

Stir the remaining ginger and a little seasoning into the yogurt. Thickly slice the pork and serve with the couscous and ginger yogurt.


Chicken & chorizo jambalaya


Ingredients

1 tbsp olive oil

2 chicken breasts, chopped

1 onion, diced

1 red pepper, thinly sliced

2 garlic cloves, crushed

75g chorizo, sliced

1 tbsp Cajun seasoning

250g long grain rice

400g can plum tomato

350ml chicken stock


Method

STEP 1

Heat 1 tbsp olive oil in a large frying pan with a lid and brown 2 chopped chicken breasts for 5-8 mins until golden.

STEP 2

Remove and set aside. Tip in the 1 diced onion and cook for 3-4 mins until soft.

STEP 3

Add 1 thinly sliced red pepper, 2 crushed garlic cloves, 75g sliced chorizo and 1 tbsp Cajun seasoning, and cook for 5 mins more.

STEP 4

Stir the chicken back in with 250g long grain rice, add the 400g can of tomatoes and 350ml chicken stock. Cover and simmer for 20-25 mins until the rice is tender.


Apple, pear & cherry compote


Ingredients

8 eating apples, peeled, cored and cut into chunks

4 medium Bramley apples, peeled, cored and cut into chunks

8 firm pears, peeled, cored and thickly sliced

6 tbsp sugar, or to taste

280g dried sour cherries (or dried cranberries)

Method

STEP 1

Put the apples and pears in a pan with the sugar and 50ml water. Bring to a simmer, then gently cook, covered, for 15 mins or so until the Bramley apple has collapsed to a purée and the eating apple and pear are tender (stir to make sure it doesn't catch on the bottom).

STEP 2

Stir in the cherries or cranberries for 1 min, taste and add a little more sugar if necessary. Can be chilled for 3-5 days. Serve with vanilla ice cream, if you like. See 'Goes well with' for ideas for using up the compote.

Pepper-crusted salmon with garlic chickpeas

Ingredients

4 skinless salmon fillets, about 150g/5oz each

2 tsp black peppercorns

1 tsp paprika

grated zest and juice 2 limes

1 tbsp olive oil

For the chickpeas

2 x 400g/14oz cans chickpeas

3 tbsp olive oil

2 garlic cloves, finely chopped

150ml vegetable stock

130g bag baby spinach


Method

STEP 1

Heat oven to 190C/fan 170C/gas 5. Put the salmon fillets in a shallow ovenproof dish in a single layer. Roughly crush the peppercorns with a pestle and mortar, or tip into a cup and crush with the end of a rolling pin. Mix with the paprika, lime zest and a little sea salt. Brush the salmon lightly with oil, then sprinkle over the pepper mix. Bake for 12-15 mins until the salmon is just cooked.

STEP 2

Meanwhile, tip the chickpeas into a colander, rinse well under cold running water, then drain. Heat the oil in a pan, add the garlic, then gently cook for 5 mins without browning. Add the chickpeas and stock, then warm through. Crush the chickpeas lightly with a potato masher, then add the spinach and stir well until the leaves are wilted. Add the lime juice and some salt and pepper, then heat through. Serve with the salmon.


Clementine, feta & winter leaf salad

Ingredients

6-8 seedless clementines

2 heads red chicory

100g watercress

1 fennel bulb, halved, cored and very finely sliced

1 red onion, halved and finely sliced

200g feta cheese, cut into cubes

small handful parsley, finely chopped

For the dressing

juice 1 clementine

juice 1 lemon

4 tbsp olive oil

1 tsp caster sugar


Method

STEP 1

Whisk the dressing ingredients in a jug, season with salt and set aside.

STEP 2

To make the salad, peel the clementines and slice whole. In a bowl, gently toss the chicory and watercress with the fennel and onion.

Place slices of clementine on opposite sides of each plate, mound a pile of leaves in the middle, then scatter over the feta. Stir the parsley through the dressing and drizzle over the salad.

Superhealthy salmon burgers

Ingredients

4 boneless, skinless salmon fillets, about 550g/1lb 4oz in total, cut into chunks

2 tbsp Thai red curry paste

thumb-size piece fresh root ginger, grated

1 tsp soy sauce

1 bunch coriander, half chopped, half leaves picked

1 tsp vegetable oil

lemon wedges, to serve

For the salad

2 carrots

half large or 1 small cucumber

2 tbsp white wine vinegar

1 tsp golden caster sugar

Method

STEP 1

Tip the salmon into a food processor with the paste, ginger, soy and chopped coriander. Pulse until roughly minced. Tip out the mix and shape into 4 burgers. Heat the oil in a non-stick frying pan, then fry the burgers for 4-5 mins on each side, turning until crisp and cooked through.

STEP 2

Meanwhile, use a swivel peeler to peel strips of carrot and cucumber into a bowl. Toss with the vinegar and sugar until the sugar has dissolved, then toss through the coriander leaves. Divide the salad between 4 plates. Serve with the burgers and rice.

Falafel burgers

Ingredients

400g can chickpeas, rinsed and drained

1 small red onion, roughly chopped

1 garlic clove, chopped

handful of flat-leaf parsley or curly parsley

1 tsp ground cumin

1 tsp ground coriander

½ tsp harissa paste or chilli powder

2 tbsp plain flour

2 tbsp sunflower oil

toasted pitta bread, to serve

200g tub tomato salsa, to serve

green salad, to serve

Method

STEP 1

Drain the chickpeas and pat dry with kitchen paper. Tip into a food processor along with the onion, garlic, parsley, cumin, coriander, harissa paste, flour and a little salt. Blend until fairly smooth, then shape into four patties with your hands.

STEP 2

Heat the sunflower oil in a non-stick frying pan, and fry the burgers for 3 mins on each side until lightly golden. Serve with the toasted pitta bread, tomato salsa and green salad.

Frozen fruit sticks with passion fruit & lime drizzle

Ingredients

100g strawberries, hulled and halved

8 seedless grapes

100g/4oz mango chunks

100g/4oz melon chunks

2 kiwi fruit, peeled and cut into chunks

100g/4oz pineapple chunks

For the drizzle

juice 2 limes

4 passion fruits, halved and seeds scraped out

1 tsp icing sugar


Method

STEP 1

Mix the drizzle ingredients in a small bowl, stirring until the sugar has dissolved. If you want the sauce to be smooth, pass it through a sieve to remove the seeds, or leave them in if you prefer.

STEP 2

Skewer the fruits onto wooden skewers and drizzle the sauce on top, reserving a little for dipping. Pop the skewers in the freezer for 45 mins, until just starting to freeze. Serve with the leftover drizzle.


Chinese chicken curry

Ingredients

4 skinless chicken breasts, cut into chunks (or use thighs or drumsticks)

2 tsp cornflour

1 onion, diced

2 tbsp rapeseed oil

1 garlic clove, crushed

2 tsp curry powder

1 tsp turmeric

½ tsp ground ginger

pinch sugar

400ml chicken stock

1 tsp soy sauce

handful frozen peas

rice to serve


Method

STEP 1

Toss the chicken pieces in the cornflour and season well. Set them aside.

STEP 2

Fry the onion in half of the oil in a wok on a low to medium heat, until it softens – about 5-6 minutes – then add the garlic and cook for a minute. Stir in the spices and sugar and cook for another minute, then add the stock and soy sauce, bring to a simmer and cook for 20 minutes. Tip everything into a blender and blitz until smooth.

STEP 3

Wipe out the pan and fry the chicken in the remaining oil until it is browned all over. Tip the sauce back into the pan and bring everything to a simmer, stir in the peas and cook for 5 minutes. Add a little water if you need to thin the sauce. Serve with rice.

Spiced shepherd's pie

Ingredients

500g pack lean minced lamb

1 onion, chopped

2 carrots, diced

2 tbsp garam masala

200ml hot stock (lamb, beef or chicken)

200g frozen peas

800g potatoes, diced

1 tsp turmeric

small bunch coriander, roughly chopped

juice half lemon, plus wedges to serve

Method

STEP 1

In a large non-stick frying pan, cook the lamb, onion and carrots, stirring often, until the lamb is browned and veg is starting to soften, about 8 mins. Add the garam masala and some seasoning and cook for a further 2 mins until fragrant. Pour in the stock, bring to the boil, tip in the peas and cook for a further 2 mins until the peas are cooked and most of the liquid has evaporated.

STEP 2

Meanwhile, cook potatoes in a large pan of salted water until just tender, about 8 mins. Drain well, return to the pan and gently stir in turmeric and coriander – try not to break up the potatoes too much.

STEP 3

Heat oven to 200C/180C fan/gas 6. Transfer the mince to a baking dish and top with the turmeric potatoes. Squeeze over the lemon juice, then bake for 30-35 mins until potatoes are golden. Serve immediately with extra lemon wedges on the side.


Sweet & sour lentil dhal with grilled aubergine

Ingredients

100g red lentils, rinsed

1 tsp turmeric

1 tbsp tamarind paste

2 tbsp vegetable oil

1 medium onion, thinly sliced

1 garlic clove, finely chopped

3cm/1¼ inch piece ginger, grated

1 tsp curry powder

1 medium aubergine, cut into 2 cm slices

cooked basmati rice, lime or mango chutney and a few coriander leaves, to serve, if you like

Method

STEP 1

Cover the lentils, turmeric and tamarind paste with 500ml water. Add some salt and boil for 15 mins or until very soft. Skim off any foam that forms on the top. Meanwhile, heat 1 tbsp of the oil and cook the onion, garlic and ginger until golden, about 5 mins.

STEP 2

Add the curry powder and cook for a further 2 mins. Pour in the lentil mixture and cook for another 10 mins.

STEP 3

Meanwhile, heat a griddle pan until very hot. Rub the remaining oil over the aubergine slices and season. Cook for 2-3 mins each side until cooked through and charred. Eat with basmati rice, lime or mango chutney and a sprinkling of coriander, if you like.

Lemon cod with basil bean mash

Ingredients

2 small bunches cherry tomatoes, on the vine

1 tbsp olive oil

chunks skinless cod or other white fish fillet

zest 1 lemon, plus juice of 0.5

240g pack frozen soya beans

1 garlic clove

bunch basil, leaves and stalks separated

100ml low-sodium chicken or vegetable stock

Method

STEP 1

Heat oven to 200C/fan 180C/gas 6. Put the tomatoes onto a baking tray, rub with a little oil and some seasoning, then roast for 5 mins until the skins are starting to split. Add the fish to the tray, top with most of the lemon zest and some more seasoning, then drizzle with a little more oil. Roast for 8-10 mins until the fish flakes easily.

STEP 2

Meanwhile, cook the beans in a pan of boiling water for 3 mins until just tender. Drain, then tip into a food processor with the rest of the oil, garlic, basil stalks, lemon juice and stock, then pulse to a thick, slightly rough purée. Season to taste.

STEP 3

Divide the tomatoes and mash between two plates, top with the cod, then scatter with basil leaves and the remaining lemon zest to serve.

Crab & sweetcorn chowder

Ingredients

1 onion, finely chopped

1 leek, green and white parts separated and sliced

2 carrots, chopped

850ml-1 litre/1.5 pints - 1.75 pints low-sodium chicken or vegetable stock

1 large potato, diced

175g/ 6oz frozen sweetcorn

170g can white crabmeat, drained

4 tbsp light crème fraîche

1 tsp chopped chives


Method

STEP 1

Put the onion, white part of the leek and carrots in a large pan and pour on a few tbsp of the stock. Cook over a medium heat for about 10 mins, stirring regularly until soft. Add a splash more stock if the vegetables start to stick.

STEP 2

Add the potato, green leek and most of the stock, and simmer for 10-15 mins, until the potato is tender. Tip in the sweetcorn and crab meat, then cook for a further 1-2 mins. Remove from the heat and stir in the crème fraîche and some seasoning. Add the rest of the stock if the soup is too thick. Sprinkle with the chives and serve with brown bread, if you like.

Lighter lemony pasta and spinach bake

Ingredients

300g/10½oz dried macaroni

200g/7oz broccoli, cut into small florets

100g/3½oz baby spinach, any thicker stems removed

2 tsp olive oil

2 spring onions, outer leaves removed, thinly sliced

1 garlic clove, thinly sliced

1 tbsp plain flour

300ml/10fl oz skimmed milk

2 bay leaves

1 tsp wholegrain mustard

1 unwaxed lemon, finely grated zest only

100g/3½oz Parmesan (or vegetarian alternative), finely grated

salt and freshly ground black pepper

mixed salad leaves dressed with a squeeze of lemon juice and 1 tsp olive oil, to serve


Method

Preheat the oven to 200C/180C Fan/Gas 6

Cook the macaroni in boiling water for 6 minutes. Add the broccoli and cook for another 2 minutes. Turn off the heat, add the spinach and leave to stand with the lid on for 2 minutes. Drain well and set aside

Heat the oil in a heavy-based frying pan. Fry the spring onions for 2 minutes. Add the garlic and fry for another 2 minutes. Add the flour and cook, stirring all the time, for 1-2 minutes. Slowly pour in the milk, add the bay leaves and season with salt and pepper. Continue simmering for 2-3 minutes, until thickened. Remove the bay leaves.

Stir in the mustard, lemon zest and three quarters of the Parmesan, then season well.

Tip the pasta and broccoli into a shallow baking dish. Pour over the sauce and mix well. Sprinkle over the remaining cheese and bake for 15-20 minutes.

Serve with the dressed salad leaves.


Low-fat chicken tikka masala


Ingredients

For the marinated chicken

500g/1lb 2oz chicken breasts, cut into bite-sized pieces

1 garlic clove, grated

75g/2½oz plain yoghurt

1 tbsp tikka spice powder

For the tikka masala sauce

1 chicken stock pot, made up with 100ml/3½fl oz boiling water

2 medium onions, sliced

2 garlic cloves, sliced

1 tsp grated fresh ginger

1½ tbsp tikka spice powder

1 x 400g tin chopped tomatoes

1 small bunch fresh coriander, chopped, plus extra for garnish

salt and freshly ground black pepper

3 tbsp plain yoghurt


To serve

300g/10½oz brown basmati rice, cooked according to packet instructions

Recipe tips


Method

For the marinated chicken, mix together all the ingredients in a bowl, cover with cling film and put in the fridge aside to marinate while you make the sauce.

For the tikka masala sauce, bring the stock to a simmer in a saucepan. Add the sliced onions, garlic and ginger. Cut a square of baking paper or greaseproof paper large enough to cover the mixture in the pan. Push it right down to cover the onions and garlic closely, cover the pan with a lid and simmer very gently for 15 minutes.

Remove the paper. The onions should be translucent and soft. Add the tikka spice powder, the tinned tomatoes and the chopped coriander and bring to the boil. Reduce the heat slightly and simmer briskly for 20-30 minutes, until the sauce is thickened. Season with salt and freshly ground black pepper then set aside to cool slightly.

Meanwhile, preheat the grill to its hottest setting. Cover a baking tray with foil, and then place the marinated chicken on the tray in a single layer. Grill the chicken for 15 minutes, or until the chicken pieces are cooked through. Give the chicken a turn halfway through cooking, to ensure it's nicely browned all over.

Using a stick blender or food processor, blend the tikka masala sauce until smooth. Return to the heat and warm through, then add the plain yoghurt. (Don't boil the sauce after you add the yoghurt or it will split.) Stir the cooked chicken pieces into the sauce and serve with brown basmati rice and a sprinkling of coriander to finish.


Healthy chicken pie


Ingredients

1 x 200g/7oz chicken breast

200ml/7fl oz semi-skimmed milk, plus a ½ tbsp extra to glaze

¼ onion, peeled

1 bay leaf

100g/3½oz reduced-calorie ready rolled puff pastry (about a 10x25cm piece)

low-calorie spray oil

2 bacon medallions, sliced into small pieces

200g/7oz button mushrooms, large ones cut in half

1 leek, chopped

1 tbsp plain flour

steamed broccoli, to serve

Recipe tips

Method

Put the chicken breast in a small pan (it needs to be a small pan so the chicken poaches in the milk). Add the milk, onion and bay leaf. Cover with a lid and simmer gently for 15 minutes, or until the chicken is cooked through.

Preheat the oven to 200C/180C Fan/Gas 6.

Divide the pastry into two equal rectangles and carefully roll them out until large enough to cover the top of two individual pie dishes. Place the upturned pie dishes on the pastry and cut around them to make the pie lids. Cut any excess pastry into strips and press them around the top edge of the pie dishes (this will help the lids stay in place as the pies bake). Cut a cross in the middle of the pastry lids and set aside.

Fry the bacon with one squirt of spray oil in a non-stick pan. When golden-brown, add the mushrooms and a tablespoon of water. Cook for 2-3 minutes then add the leeks. Cook for about 5 minutes breaking up the leeks as they soften.

Remove the chicken from the poaching milk. Strain and reserve the milk and chop the chicken into bite-sized pieces.

Stir the chicken into the vegetables. Add the flour and stir well. Cook for 2 minutes, then add the strained poaching milk stirring well to incorporate. Continue to cook for 2-3 minutes, or until the sauce has thickened just a little. Divide between the pie dishes.

Brush the pastry edges with a little milk and add the pie lids. Brush all over with more milk. Bake for 25 minutes, or until the pastry lid is golden-brown. Serve immediately with steamed broccoli.


Chicken and vegetable balti


Ingredients

calorie controlled cooking oil spray

1 medium onion, thinly sliced

4 chicken thighs, boned and skinned

1 red pepper, deseeded and cut into 3cm/1in chunks

1 yellow pepper, deseeded and cut into 3cm/1in chunks

1 tbsp cornflour

150g/5½oz fat-free natural yogurt

1 tbsp medium or mild curry powder

2 garlic cloves, thinly sliced

227g/8oz tin chopped tomatoes

3 heaped tbsp finely chopped fresh coriander, plus extra to garnish

freshly ground black pepper


Method

Spray a large, deep, non-stick frying pan or wok with oil and place over a medium heat. Add the onion and cook for five minutes, stirring regularly until well softened and lightly browned.

Meanwhile, trim all the visible fat off the chicken thighs, cut each one into four pieces and season with black pepper.

Add the chicken and peppers into the pan with the onion and cook for three minutes, turning occasionally.

Meanwhile, in a small bowl, mix the cornflour with 2 tablespoons cold water and stir in the yoghurt until thoroughly mixed.

Sprinkle the curry powder over the chicken and vegetables, add the garlic and cook for 30 seconds.

Tip the tomatoes into the pan, add the yoghurt mixture, 150ml/3½fl oz of water and coriander.

Bring to a gentle simmer and cook for 20-25 minutes, stirring occasionally until the chicken is tender and the sauce is thick. Season with freshly ground black pepper to taste and garnish with coriander.

Hearty vegetable soup

Ingredients

calorie controlled cooking oil spray

1 medium onion, sliced

2 garlic cloves, thinly sliced

2 celery sticks, trimmed and thinly sliced

2 medium carrots or 2 yellow peppers, cut into 2cm/1in chunks

400g/14oz tin chopped tomatoes

1 vegetable stock cube

1 tsp dried mixed herbs

400g/14oz tin butter beans, drained and rinsed

1 head young spring greens (approximately 125g/4½oz), trimmed and sliced

sea salt and freshly ground black pepper

Method

Spray a large non-stick saucepan with oil and cook the onion, garlic, celery and carrots or peppers gently for 10 minutes, stirring regularly until softened.

Add 750ml/26fl oz water and the chopped tomatoes. Crumble over the stock cube and stir in the dried herbs. Bring to the boil, then reduce the heat to a simmer and cook for 20 minutes.

Season the soup with salt and pepper and add the spring greens and butterbeans. Return to a gentle simmer and cook for a further 3-4 minutes or until the greens are softened. Season to taste and serve in deep bowls.


Healthy chilli con carne


Ingredients

low-calorie cooking spray

450g/1lb extra lean minced beef (5% fat)

1 large red onion, finely chopped

3 tsp finely grated garlic

1 courgette, cut into 1cm/½in pieces

1 aubergine, cut into 1cm/½in pieces

1 red pepper, deseeded and cut into 1cm/½in pieces

2 tsp ground cumin

1 tsp sweet smoked paprika

½ tsp ground cinnamon

1 tsp hot chilli powder

400g tin red kidney beans in chilli sauce

400g tin chopped tomatoes

4 tbsp tomato purée

200ml/7fl oz beef stock

200g/7oz brown basmati rice

salt and freshly ground black pepper

4 tbsp fat-free natural yoghurt and chopped fresh coriander, to serve

Method

Spray a large frying pan with cooking spray. Add the beef and stir-fry over a high heat for 5–6 minutes, or until lightly browned.

Add the onion, garlic, courgette, aubergine and red pepper and stir-fry for a further 3–4 minutes. Add the cumin, smoked paprika, cinnamon and chilli powder and stir-fry for 1–2 minutes.

Add the kidney beans, tomatoes, tomato purée and stock and season well. Bring to the boil, then reduce the heat to a simmer, cover and cook for 25–30 minutes, stirring occasionally.

Uncover, stir and cook over a medium heat for 10 minutes.

Meanwhile, cook the rice according to the packet instructions.

Ladle the chilli over the rice in warmed bowls and serve immediately, with a dollop of fat-free yogurt and some chopped coriander.


Tofu Thai green curry


Ingredients

2 shallots, thinly sliced

½ tsp sesame oil

1 green finger chilli, finely chopped (optional)

2 tbsp Thai green curry paste (seek out a vegetarian version if required)

300ml/10fl oz hot vegetable stock

200g/7oz lighter coconut milk

1 tsp Thai fish sauce or light soy sauce

1 medium aubergine, cut into 2cm/1in chunks

2 kaffir lime leaves

200g/7oz tofu, cut into 1.5cm/½in squares

½ green pepper, cut into thin slices

50g/1¾oz mangetout

50g/1¾oz baby corn, halved or cut into quarters, depending on size juice of 1 lime, plus lime wedges to serve

handful finely chopped fresh coriander, to serve

150g/5½oz basmati rice, to serve


Method

Fry the shallots in the oil over a medium heat for 2–3 minutes. Add the chilli and fry for 1 minute. Stir in the curry paste and fry for 1 minute.

Pour in the hot stock, coconut milk and Thai fish sauce (if using) and bring to the boil. Reduce the heat and simmer for 5 minutes.

Add the aubergine and lime leaves and cook for 10 minutes.

Meanwhile, cook the rice according to the packet instructions.

Add the tofu and green pepper to the curry and cook with the lid off for 3 minutes. Add the mangetout and baby corn (if using) and squeeze in the lime juice. Cook for 3 minutes.

Serve the curry with the rice, sprinkled with coriander and with a wedge of lime.


Gammon and chips with pineapple and greens


Ingredients

400g/14oz floury potatoes

1 tsp olive oil, plus spray oil for frying

salt and freshly ground black pepper

2 slices fresh pineapple

250g/9oz lean gammon steak, fat trimmed

150g/5½oz Brussels sprouts, trimmed and quartered


Method

Preheat the oven to 220C/200C

Scrub the potatoes well, then half-peel them, leaving some of the nutritious skin on for extra flavour. Cut into fairly thin chips – about 1cm thick which will crisp more easily. Put into a saucepan and cover with cold water. Cover the pan, bring the water to the boil over a high heat and cook the potatoes for 3 minutes. Drain and allow to steam dry for 2-3 minutes.

Put the olive oil into a baking tray and heat in the oven for a minute. Add the drained, dried chips to the hot oil, giving the tray a gentle shake to separate the chips. They should be in a single layer. Season with a little salt and black pepper, then bake for 30-40 minutes, turning the chips halfway through cooking to move the outer chips to the middle and vice versa so they all crisp evenly.

Meanwhile, spray a frying pan lightly with spray oil. Heat the pan over a medium-high heat and, when hot, add the pineapple rings. Fry for 2 minutes per side, turning regularly, until the slices are golden-brown and caramelised. Set aside.

Reduce the heat to medium, spray the gammon steak lightly with spray oil and fry in the same pan for 4-5 minutes, turning regularly, until the steak is nicely browned and cooked through. Set aside.

Return the pan to the heat and add the Brussels sprouts. Stir-fry the sprouts for 3 minutes, adding a splash of water if necessary, until they are bright green but still retain a bit of bite.

Serve the gammon steaks with the pineapple on top, with the stir-fried sprouts and chips alongside.

Light smoked haddock fish pie

Ingredients

1 tbsp olive oil

1 leek, sliced

30g/1oz flour

300ml/½ pint milk

125g/4½oz prawns, cooked and peeled

salt and freshly ground black pepper

4 x 110g/4oz smoked haddock fillets

3 large potatoes, peeled, par-boiled and sliced

Method

Pre-heat oven to 200C/400F

Heat the oil in a pan over a medium heat. Add the leeks and fry for 2-3 minutes, until soft.

Add the flour, stir well and cook for 1-2 minutes.

Remove the pan from the heat and gradually stir in the milk. Return to the heat and cook, stirring well, until the sauce has thickened. Simmer gently for five minutes.

Stir in the prawns and season with salt and pepper.

Place half the sauce into a pie dish. Place the haddock fillets on top, then spoon over the remaining sauce.

Top with the sliced potatoes and season with some more freshly ground black pepper.

Place the dish on a baking sheet and bake for 35-40 minutes, until the potatoes are golden and the fish is completely cooked through.

Mexican bean stew

Ingredients

low-calorie cooking spray

1 onion, thinly sliced

2 garlic cloves, crushed

1 yellow pepper, deseeded and cut into 3cm/1in chunks

½ tsp hot chilli powder

1 tsp ground cumin

1 tsp ground coriander

400g tin chopped tomatoes

2 tbsp tomato purée

400g tin mixed beans, drained and rinsed

125g/4½oz wholegrain long-grain rice, to serve

100g/3½oz fat-free Greek yoghurt, to serve

1 lime, cut into wedges, to serve

salt and freshly ground black pepper

For the salsa

1 tomato, roughly chopped

4 tbsp roughly chopped freshly coriander

2 spring onions, thinly sliced


Method

Spray a large frying pan with oil and place over a medium heat. Add the onion and garlic and cook gently for three minutes, stirring regularly. Add the pepper and cook for two minutes.

Stir in the spices and cook for a few seconds, then add the tomatoes, tomato purée and mixed beans. Pour over 300ml/10fl oz cold water and bring to a gentle simmer. Season with a little salt and lots of ground black pepper and cook for 30 minutes, stirring occasionally until thick.

Meanwhile half-fill a medium saucepan with water and bring to the boil. Add the rice and return to the boil. Cook for 25 minutes, or until tender, stirring occasionally.

To make the salsa, mix the tomato, coriander and spring onions together in a bowl.

Drain the rice and divide between two plates. Spoon the beans over and scatter with the salsa. Serve with the yoghurt and lime wedges.

Healthy scrambled eggs

Ingredients

8 midi vine tomatoes, halved

low-calorie cooking spray

3 large free-range eggs

35g/1¼oz smoked salmon, roughly chopped

1 tbsp chopped chives

25g/1oz fresh watercress, to serve

freshly ground black pepper


Method

Season the tomatoes with pepper. Heat a pan sprayed with cooking spray oil over a medium heat, add the tomatoes and cook for 2-3 minutes, until softened, stirring from time to time but not breaking up the tomatoes.

Meanwhile, beat the eggs in a bowl with some pepper. Stir in the salmon and chives and pour into a saucepan.

Cook very gently for 3-4 minutes, stirring slowly, until the eggs are softly scrambled. Remove from the heat and stir for a few seconds.

Divide the tomatoes between two plates and serve with the scrambled eggs and watercress


Cinnamon porridge with grated pear


Ingredients

60g/2¼oz jumbo porridge oats

¼ tsp ground cinnamon, plus a little to sprinkle

300ml/10fl oz semi-skimmed milk

1 ripe medium pear

1 wedge lemon

Method

Put the oats and cinnamon in a non-stick saucepan with the milk and cook over a low-medium heat for 4-5 minutes, stirring constantly until rich and creamy. Pour into two deep bowls.

Coarsely grate the pear, and place on top of the porridge. Squeeze over the lemon juice and sprinkle with a tiny pinch of ground cinnamon.

Peanut butter and raspberry porridge recipe

Ingredients

1 oats sachet

180ml semi-skimmed milk

1 tbsp crunchy peanut butter

50g frozen raspberries

½ tbsp chia seeds

Method

Make the oats to pack instructions. Spoon into a bowl.

Top the porridge with the peanut butter and raspberries, then lightly swirl with a dessert spoon, allowing the raspberries soften in the warm porridge.

Sprinkle with the chia seeds to serve.

Healthy pancakes with lemon cream cheese recipe

Ingredients

100g light cream cheese

1 lemon, juiced and finely zested, plus extra to garnish

200g wholemeal plain flour

1 tsp baking powder

small handful basil leaves, chopped

small handful parsley, chopped

2 eggs, separated

200ml semi-skimmed milk

butter, for greasing

1 avocado, quartered and sliced

150g cherry tomatoes, halved


Method

In a bowl, combine the cream cheese with the lemon zest and juice. Season with freshly cracked black pepper and set aside until needed.

Sift the flour, baking powder, herbs and ¼ tsp salt into a large mixing bowl and make a well in the centre.

Add the egg yolks and half the milk. Using a fork, gently stir to combine, drawing in the flour from the sides of the bowl. Add the remaining milk and continue mixing to form a completely smooth batter.

In a separate bowl, whisk the egg whites, using an electric whisk, until stiff peaks form. Using a large, metal spoon, gently fold the egg whites into the batter, being careful not to knock the air out.

Put a large, nonstick frying pan over a medium-high heat and lightly brush with a little butter to grease. Spoon 4 generous tbsp of batter into the pan to make 4 separate pancakes – space them out as they will spread a little. Cook for 1 min, until bubbles rise to the surface, then turn and cook for a further 30 seconds–1 min. Transfer to a warm plate, covered with a tea towel. Repeat to make 16 pancakes.

To serve, arrange 4 pancakes on each plate with some sliced avocado and tomatoes. Top with a dollop of the lemon cream cheese and scatter with a little extra lemon zest.


Mexican-style baked eggs recipe


Ingredients

4 corn tortillas, each cut into 8 triangles

1 tbsp olive oil

1 red onion, sliced

2 garlic cloves, crushed

400g tin Grower's Harvest red kidney beans, drained and rinsed

400g tin chopped tomatoes

4 eggs

100g low-fat Greek-style yogurt

1 lime, 1/2 juiced, 1/2 cut into wedges

5g fresh coriander, leaves picked

1 small avocado, diced


Method

Preheat the oven to gas 7, 220°C, fan 200°C. Put the tortilla triangles on a large baking tray, spaced apart, and set aside.

Heat the oil in a large, ovenproof frying pan over a medium heat. Fry the onion for 5 mins, then add the garlic and fry for 1 min. Add the kidney beans and fry for 2 mins, then add the tomatoes and ½ tin of water.

Bring to the boil, then reduce the heat and simmer for 10 mins. Make 4 indents in the sauce and crack an egg into each one. Cook for 5 mins until the eggs are starting to set. Transfer the pan to the oven and put the tortillas on the shelf below. Bake for 5-7 mins until the eggs are set and the tortillas are golden.

Meanwhile, mix the yogurt with the lime juice. To serve, scatter the coriander and avocado over the eggs and serve with the crispy tortillas, lime wedges and yogurt.


Roasted spiced broccoli soup recipe


Ingredients

1 medium broccoli (about 400g), florets and stalks roughly chopped

1 tbsp vegetable oil

2 tsp ground coriander

2 tsp ground cumin

pinch ground cayenne pepper

1 large onion, roughly chopped

2 celery sticks, roughly chopped

½ x 30g pack fresh parsley, stalks finely chopped and leaves picked

1 large baking potato (about 200g), peeled and cut into 2cm chunks

½ vegetable stock pot, dissolved in 800ml boiling water

200ml almond milk

½ lemon, juiced

100g baby leaf spinach

2 tbsp dry roasted peanuts, roughly chopped


Method

Preheat the oven to gas 7, 220°C, fan 200°C. On a large baking tray toss the broccoli, ½ tbsp oil and ground spices together until well combined. Roast in the oven for 20 mins until the broccoli is lightly charred and starting to soften.

Meanwhile, heat the remaining ½ tbsp oil in a large saucepan over a medium heat, add the onion, celery, parsley stalks and potato, cover and cook for 5 mins, stirring occasionally, until the onion has started to soften. Increase the heat to high, add the stock, re-cover and boil for 10 mins until the potato is soft. Add the roasted broccoli, almond milk, lemon juice and spinach to the pan, bring to the boil and simmer for 2 mins until the spinach has wilted then blend with a stick blender until smooth.

Divide the soup between 4 bowls and serve topped with the peanuts, the parsley leaves and a pinch of chilli flakes. This soup freezes well and will keep in the fridge for up to 3 days.

## Spiced carrot & lentil soup

### Ingredients

2 tsp cumin seeds

pinch chilli flakes

2 tbsp olive oil

600g carrots, washed and coarsely grated (no need to peel)

140g split red lentils

1l hot vegetable stock (from a cube is fine)

125ml milk (to make it dairy-free, see 'try' below)

plain yogurt and naan bread, to serve

### Method

STEP 1

Heat a large saucepan and dry-fry 2 tsp cumin seeds and a pinch of chilli flakes for 1 min, or until they start to jump around the pan and release their aromas.

STEP 2

Scoop out about half with a spoon and set aside. Add 2 tbsp olive oil, 600g coarsely grated carrots, 140g split red lentils, 1l hot vegetable stock and 125ml milk to the pan and bring to the boil.

STEP 3

Simmer for 15 mins until the lentils have swollen and softened.

STEP 4

Whizz the soup with a stick blender or in a food processor until smooth (or leave it chunky if you prefer).

STEP 5

Season to taste and finish with a dollop of plain yogurt and a sprinkling of the reserved toasted spices. Serve with warmed naan breads.

Healthy beef stew

Ingredients

1 onion, sliced

1 garlic clove, sliced

2 tbsp olive oil

300g pack beef stir-fry strips, or use beef steak, thinly sliced

1 yellow pepper, deseeded and thinly sliced

400g can chopped tomato

sprig rosemary, chopped

handful pitted olives

Method

STEP 1

In a large saucepan, cook onion and garlic in olive oil for 5 mins until softened and turning golden. Tip in the beef strips, pepper, tomatoes and rosemary, then bring to the boil. Simmer for 15 mins until the meat is cooked through, adding some boiling water if needed. Stir through the olives and serve with mash or polenta.

Celery soup

Ingredients

2 tbsp olive oil

300g celery, sliced, with tough strings removed

1 garlic clove, peeled

200g potatoes, peeled and cut into chunks

500ml vegetable stock

100ml milk

crusty bread, to serve


Method

STEP 1

Heat the oil in a large saucepan over a medium heat, tip in the celery, garlic and potatoes and coat in the oil. Add a splash of water and a big pinch of salt and cook, stirring regularly for 15 mins, adding a little more water if the veg begins to stick.

STEP 2

Pour in the vegetable stock and bring to the boil, then turn the heat down and simmer for 20 mins further, until the potatoes are falling apart and the celery is soft. Use a stick blender to purée the soup, then pour in the milk and blitz again. Season to taste. Serve with crusty bread.


Pan-fried venison with blackberry sauce

Ingredients

1 tbsp olive oil

2 thick venison steaks, or 4 medallions

1 tbsp balsamic vinegar

150ml beef stock (made with 2 tsp Knorr Touch of Taste beef concentrate)

2 tbsp redcurrant jelly

1 garlic clove, crushed

85g fresh or frozen blackberry

Method

STEP 1

Heat the oil in a frying pan, cook the venison for 5 mins, then turn over and cook for 3-5 mins more, depending on how rare you like it and the thickness of the meat (cook for 5-6 mins on each side for well done). Lift the meat from the pan and set aside to rest.

STEP 2

Add the balsamic vinegar to the pan, then pour in the stock, redcurrant jelly and garlic. Stir over quite a high heat to blend everything together, then add the blackberries and carry on cooking until they soften. Serve with the venison, celeriac mash (see below) and broccoli.

Red lentil, chickpea & chilli soup

Ingredients

2 tsp cumin seeds

large pinch chilli flakes

1 tbsp olive oil

1 red onion, chopped

140g red split lentils

850ml vegetable stock or water

400g can tomatoes, whole or chopped

200g can chickpeas or ½ a can, drained and rinsed (freeze leftovers)

small bunch coriander, roughly chopped (save a few leaves, to serve)

4 tbsp 0% Greek yogurt, to serve

Method

STEP 1

Heat a large saucepan and dry-fry 2 tsp cumin seeds and a large pinch
of chilli flakes for 1 min, or until they start to jump around the pan and
release their aromas.

STEP 2

Add 1 tbsp olive oil and 1 chopped red onion, and cook for 5 mins.

STEP 3

Stir in 140g red split lentils, 850ml vegetable stock or water and a 400g can tomatoes, then bring to the boil. Simmer for 15 mins until the lentils have softened.

STEP 4

Whizz the soup with a stick blender or in a food processor until it is a rough purée, pour back into the pan and add a 200g can drained and rinsed chickpeas

STEP 5

Heat gently, season well and stir in a small bunch of chopped coriander, reserving a few leaves to serve. Finish with 4 tbsp 0% Greek yogurt and extra coriander leaves.

Braised sea bass with spinach

Ingredients

2 red peppers, halved, deseeded

2 tbsp extra-virgin olive oil, plus extra for drizzling

2 shallots, chopped

1 garlic clove, finely chopped

250g cherry or baby plum tomato, halved

small handful capers

12 large black olives, stoned and roughly chopped

20 basil leaves

50ml white wine

100ml/3½ fl oz tomato juice

2 whole sea bass, about 600-700g/1lb 5oz-1lb-9oz each, gutted, scaled and cleaned (get your fishmonger to do this)

large knob butter

250g bag spinach


Method

STEP 1

Heat the grill to high. Put the peppers, skin side up, on a baking tray, then pop them under the hot grill for about 10 mins until the skins blister and blacken. Drop them into a bowl, cover with some cling film and leave until cool enough to handle. Peel away and discard the skins, then roughly chop the peppers.

STEP 2

Heat the oil over a low-ish heat in a sturdy roasting tin or in a shallow pan that has a lid and is large enough to fit both fish. Throw in the shallots and garlic and sweat briefly until soft. Stir in the tomatoes, peppers, capers, olives and half the basil leaves, then sweat for a few mins until the tomatoes soften. Pour in the wine and tomato juice. Stir and gently simmer for 10-15 mins, adding a splash of water if the sauce becomes a bit dry.

STEP 3

While the sauce is simmering, slash each side of the fish a few times. When the sauce is ready lay the fish on top, season if you want to and cover with a lid (cover with foil if you are using a roasting tray). Leave to cook on a low heat for 12-15 mins until the flesh feels firm when pressed.

STEP 4

While the fish is cooking, melt the butter in a large pan, then fry the spinach until wilted, season if you like and divide the spinach between two serving dishes. Lift the fish carefully from the pan and place on top of the spinach, neatly drizzle some of the sauce round the fish, scatter the remaining basil on top and drizzle everything with extra-virgin olive oil. Serve with some ribbon shaped pasta, like tagliatelle or pappardelle, with the remaining sauce in a bowl or side dish.

Caramelised carrots & onions

Ingredients

500g carrot, peeled and cut into long chunks

50g butter

1 tbsp olive oil

8 red onions, peeled and quartered with root intact

3 sprigs thyme

1 tbsp soft brown sugar

3 tbsp red wine

1 tbsp good-quality balsamic vinegar

Method

STEP 1

Blanch carrots in a pan of boiling salted water for 3 mins, drain well, then pat dry. In a large pan, melt the butter and oil, then fry the carrots, onions and thyme over a low heat for 30 mins until golden.

STEP 2

Stir in the sugar and red wine and bubble for a few mins to boil off the alcohol. Add the vinegar, then continue to cook until syrupy, about 5 mins. Remove the sprigs of thyme and serve. Make up to 2 days ahead, stored in a covered container. Tip back into a pan and reheat or use a microwave.

Chicken jalfrezi

Ingredients

For the sauce

½ large onion, roughly chopped

2 garlic cloves, chopped

1 green chilli, finely chopped

vegetable oil, for frying

400g can plum tomatoes

1 tbsp ground coriander

1 tbsp ground cumin

1 tsp turmeric

For the meat & veg

2-3 chicken breasts, diced

1 tsp ground cumin

1 tsp ground coriander

1 tsp turmeric

½ large onion, sliced

1 red pepper, chopped

2 red chillies, finely chopped (optional)

2 tsp garam masala

handful of fresh, chopped coriander leaves

cooked basmati rice or naan bread to serve


Method

STEP 1

Take 2-3 diced chicken breasts and coat in 1 tsp cumin, 1 tsp coriander and 1 tsp turmeric then leave it to marinate in the fridge while you make the sauce.

STEP 2

To make the sauce, fry ½ roughly chopped large onion, 2 chopped garlic cloves and 1 finely chopped green chilli in a large pan with a little vegetable oil, for around 5 mins, until browned.

STEP 3

Add 300ml water to the onion mixture and simmer for around 20 minutes.

STEP 4

Meanwhile, put a 400g can plum tomatoes in a food processor and give it a good whizz (aim for a smooth consistency).

STEP 5

Heat another large pan and gently fry 1 tbsp coriander, 1 tbsp cumin and 1 tsp turmeric in a splash of oil for about a minute. Add the tomatoes to this pan and simmer for around 10 minutes.

STEP 6

Next, whizz your onion mixture in the food processor and add it to the spiced tomato sauce. Season generously, stir, then simmer for 20 minutes. You can make large batches of this sauce and freeze it for later use.

STEP 7

Fry the marinated chicken in vegetable oil and stir continuously. After a few minutes, turn down the heat and add the remaining ½ sliced onion, 1 chopped red pepper and 2 finely chopped red chillies. Stir until the onions and pepper soften.

STEP 8

Add the sauce you prepared earlier to the cooked chicken and simmer for around 10-20 minutes, adding a splash of water if it gets too thick.

STEP 9

Just before you dish it up, stir in 2 tsp garam masala and handful of chopped coriander leaves. Serve with basmati rice or naan bread.

Turkey-stuffed tomatoes with wholewheat couscous salad recipe

Ingredients

2 large beef tomatoes

2 tsp olive oil

½ red onion, finely diced

2 garlic cloves, crushed

200g 2% fat turkey breast mince

1 tbsp sundried tomato purée

10g fresh basil, chopped

50g wholewheat couscous

½ lemon, juiced

10g fresh flat-leaf parsley, chopped

10g fresh mint, chopped

50g sugarsnap peas, trimmed and sliced diagonally

½ cucumber, shaved into strips with a veg peeler

Method

Preheat the oven to gas 6, 200ºC, fan 180ºC. Carefully slice the tops of the beef tomatoes off and set aside. Using a small sharp knife, cut out the flesh and seeds from the inside of the tomatoes to hollow out. Set aside the hollow tomatoes in a baking dish. Chop the inner tomato and reserve for the couscous.

Heat 1 tsp of the oil in a nonstick frying pan over a medium heat. Cook half the onion and the garlic for 5 mins until beginning to soften. Add the turkey mince and cook for 3-5 mins until browned.

Add the sundried tomato purée and cook for 1 min. Remove from the heat and stir through half the basil. Spoon the mixture into the tomatoes, cover with the tomato 'lid' and bake for 15 mins.

For the salad, put the couscous in a large bowl, pour over 75ml boiling water and cover. Let stand for 5 mins to absorb the water, then fluff with a fork.

Stir through the lemon juice and remaining olive oil. Mix through the rest of the basil along with the parsley, mint and the reserved tomato flesh. Loosely stir through the sugarsnap peas and cucumber ribbons.

To serve, carefully lift a stuffed tomato onto each plate and serve with the couscous salad.

Turkey meatball laksa recipe

Ingredients

500g pack turkey breast mince

3cm piece ginger, peeled and grated

15g fresh coriander, finely chopped, plus extra to serve

1 lime, ½ zested and juiced, the rest cut into wedges

1 tbsp vegetable oil

4 tbsp Thai red curry paste

200ml lighter coconut milk

½ reduced-salt chicken stock cube, made up to 800ml

80g Tenderstem broccoli, trimmed

80g mangetout

2 pak choi, quartered

250g wholewheat noodles

2 spring onions, finely sliced

1 red chilli, finely sliced

IF YOU DON'T HAVE ANY LIMES, TRY A LEMON INSTEAD


Method

Combine the turkey mince, ginger, coriander and lime zest in a mixing bowl. Roll into 16 balls and set aside on a tray.

Heat the vegetable oil in a large saucepan over a medium heat and fry the curry paste for 2-3 mins until aromatic. Pour in the coconut milk and chicken stock and bring to a simmer. Add the meatballs and cook for 5 mins, then add the vegetables; simmer for 3-4 mins or until just tender.

Meanwhile, cook the noodles to pack instructions, then drain and briefly rinse under cold water. Season the broth with the lime juice, then divide the noodles between 4 bowls. Spoon over the broth, meatballs and vegetables and serve with the lime wedges, spring onions, chilli and extra coriander.

Smoky chipotle adzuki bean chilli recipe


Ingredients

2 tbsp olive oil

1 red onion, roughly chopped

1 celery stick, roughly chopped

2 red peppers, cut into chunks

2 garlic cloves, crushed

15g fresh coriander, leaves picked, stalks finely chopped

1 tsp sweet smoked paprika

2 tsp chipotle chilli paste

400g tin plum tomatoes

400g tin adzuki beans

400g tin cannellini beans

1 lime, cut into wedges

long-grain and wild rice, to serve (optional)

fat-free natural yogurt, to serve (optional)

IF YOU DON'T HAVE RED ONIONS, TRY USING WHITE, BROWN OR
SPRING ONIONS

Method

Heat the oil in a large flameproof casserole dish or saucepan over a medium heat and fry the onion, celery and peppers for 10 mins or until softened, stirring regularly. Add the garlic and coriander stalks; fry for 2 mins more, stirring regularly.

Stir in the paprika and chipotle chilli paste; fry for 1 min. Add the tinned tomatoes, breaking them up with the back of the wooden spoon, then add the beans along with the liquid in the tins. Bring to the boil, then reduce the heat to low and simmer for 25 mins until thick and rich. Season with pepper to taste.

Spoon into bowls with rice and natural yogurt, if you like. Scatter over the coriander leaves and serve with lime wedges to squeeze over.


White fish with bean mash recipe


Ingredients

2 x 265g packs basa fillets

5 tsp olive oil, plus extra for drizzling

2 lemons, 1 zested and juiced, 1 sliced

1 garlic clove, crushed

2 x 400g tins cannellini beans, drained

100ml vegetable stock

2 Little Gem lettuces, quartered lengthways

1 red onion, thinly sliced

30g pack fresh flat-leaf parsley, roughly chopped


Method

Preheat the oven to gas 6, 200°C, fan 180°C. Put the fish on a baking tray lined with nonstick baking paper. Pour over 3 tsp oil and the lemon juice; season with pepper. Bake for 15-17 mins until the fish is cooked through and flakes easily.

Meanwhile, heat 1 tsp oil in a saucepan over a low heat. Add the garlic, cook for 1 min until fragrant, then add the beans and stock. Simmer for 5 mins to heat through. Add the lemon zest, season and transfer to a food processor. Blitz until smooth, then cover and set aside.

Preheat a griddle pan to very hot. Brush the cut sides of the lettuce with the remaining oil; season with pepper. Cook the lettuce over a medium heat for 5 mins each side until charred and tender.

Put the onion in a heatproof bowl, pour over enough boiling water to cover, leave for 30 secs, then drain, rinse with cold water and drain again. Stir most of the parsley into the bean mash; divide between 4 plates. Serve with the lemon slices, fish, onion and lettuce, drizzled with a little oil and sprinkled with the remaining parsley.


Low-Carb Peanut Butter Cookies

Ingredients

 1 cup creamy peanut butter (no added salt and sugar)

1 large egg

⅔ cup erythritol (powdered)

½ teaspoon baking soda

½ teaspoon vanilla extract

Instructions

Preheat oven to 350°F (180°C) and line a cookie sheet with parchment paper. Set aside.

Skip this step if using a confectioner's low-carb sweetener. Add the erythritol to a Nutribulletor blender and blend until powdered. Set aside.

Add all of the ingredients into a medium mixing bowl and mix until a smooth, glossy dough forms.

1 cup creamy peanut butter,1 large egg,⅔ cup erythritol,½ teaspoon baking soda,½ teaspoon vanilla extract

Roll about 2 tablespoons of cookie dough between your palms to form a ball, then transfer to the prepared cookie sheet. Repeat until all dough has been used. You should end up with 12-14 cookies.

Use a fork to flatten the cookies, creating a criss-cross pattern across the top.

Bake the cookies for 12-15 minutes.

Remove from the oven and allow to cool for 25 minutes on the baking sheet, then transfer to a cooling rack for another 15 minutes.

Greens, sweet potatoAND FRIED EGG BOWL

Ingredients

2 cups lettuce of choice

Olive oil (1 tbsp, plus more for drizzling)

1 sweet potato, cubed

1 large egg

½ avocado

½ cup microgreens

Salt, to taste

Juice of ½ lemon

Directions

Preheat the oven to 375 degrees F and line a baking pan with parchment paper. Lay the cubed sweet potato onto the pan and drizzle with olive oil and a sprinkle of salt. Roast in the oven for 35 to 45 minutes.

Next, heat 1 tbsp oil in a pan on the stove over medium heat. Crack the egg into the pan and fry for 2 to 3 minutes, until crispy.

Assemble the salad by adding lettuce, microgreens, roasted sweet potato, fried egg, and avocado to a bowl. Drizzle with oil, lemon juice, and salt.

## Conclusions

The Diabetic Delight Cookbook offers a delicious and healthy approach to managing diabetes through food. By focusing on fresh, whole ingredients and a balance of nutrients, this cookbook provides tasty and satisfying recipes that can help individuals with diabetes maintain a healthy diet and lifestyle.

Throughout the chapters, readers are guided on how to make healthy food choices, balance their blood sugar levels, and enjoy a wide range of flavors and textures. With a variety of recipes from breakfast to dinner, snacks and desserts, this cookbook shows that healthy eating can still be enjoyable.

The emphasis on simple ingredients and easy-to-follow instructions ensures that even those who are new to cooking can create tasty, healthy meals in their own kitchens. Whether it's a savory casserole or a sweet treat, the recipes in this cookbook offer a guilt-free way to enjoy delicious food while managing diabetes.